HOW TO MANAGE YOUR APPETITE AND LIVE A PROSPEROUS LIFE

Eric Johnson

CONTENTS

Introduction

Do you eat to satisfy your taste buds or only to stimulate your appetite? Or do you eat in an effort to exert more control over your life?

This eBook demonstrates how improving your diet alone can significantly improve your quality of life.

CHAPTER 1

Why Do We Have Health Issues Now?

The world is far less healthy than it was twenty years ago. A large portion of this is related to peoples' altered eating patterns.

In the past, individuals would never have imagined picking up the first packet of junk food they could find to feed their faces. These days, we act in such a casual manner. When someone says, "I'm hungry," they typically mean, "I want a hamburger or a frankfurter, perhaps with chips and one soda." "Let's go out and party," in this context, refers to "let's go out and drink till we can't stand up on our own and intersperse the drinks with as much synthetic-laden want to be Chinese food as we can get." Furthermore, saying "I'm on a diet" actually means "I'm taking a chemically based tablet that will snuff out my hunger and deprive my body of vitamins."

The fact that we are currently dealing with so many health issues is really no surprise. What we eat influences our health. The unfortunate state in which we find ourselves is not an issue that just affects one person; it affects everyone. The entire world is eating improperly. Check out these details: In the US, 6 out of every 10 people are overweight, and by 2015, that percentage will rise to 8 out of every 10. Due to different obesity-related problems, the US, the world's largest economy, spends close to $147 billion annually on healthcare. And the majority of the world's so-called industrialized countries are in the same condition.

Just think about how much wealthier the US would have been if it hadn't had to deal with this issue, if you only take into account this one fact. The US reserves would have had an additional $150 billion year that they might have used for development. There would likely have been more research being done, more schools and colleges (we know there are never enough of them), improvements to people's lifestyles, and so much more. With that much money, the US could provide a year's worth of food for three underdeveloped nations in Africa.

Are we really considering this? We're not. You probably have a packet of Frito Lays on the side as you read this eBook. Do you realize that instead of feeding you some of the most harmful chemicals known to mankind, that package might have fed a malnourished child in Rwanda?

But it goes beyond simply being charitable. It also pertains to us.

Yes, we must be self-centered. Aren't these concerning health statistics a sign that our time is numbered? We most certainly aren't eating properly. We must be ready for whatever excess baggage that obesity and the other health issues it leaves behind may bring.

CHAPTER 2
Providing a Fix

There is indeed grounds for concern. Our dietary practices are driving us to despair. But there is still hope. We still have time to cut costs and seek other answers.

So far, we have made terrible eating mistakes. Things won't get better unless we assess the circumstance and take control of the situation.

The first step is being conscious. We must educate ourselves on the best and worst meals to eat. We must return to school (figuratively speaking, of course) to learn what nutrients your body actually needs and in what quantities. The next step is to create a diet plan for our family and ourselves so that we may eat healthier. We must consume less of the unhealthy foods —carbohydrates, fats, and sugars, which we don't really want—and more of the ones that can improve our health.

I realize that this sounds very preachy. But that is the only respite we\shave received. We will never get better if we continue to eat Oreos.

Still, there is hope. There are numerous things that are equally as tasty as those horrible junk foods, but we are still unaware of them, therefore there is yet hope. These are the foods we don't yet know about, either because we don't like them or because we don't know how to make them, but a good health cookbook may help you learn about the many fun methods to cook healthily.

You can create some extremely tasty healthy recipes even with the same type of diet you now follow. All of that is definitely feasible. You can significantly alter your eating patterns while also taking care of your palate.

The truth is that the weight loss industry has significantly contributed to the decline of the advanced human race.

The media never explains to you how you can actually take matters into your own hands because they need to keep selling their Atkins, Jenny Craig, Zone, and Medifast products. They present us with flashy before-and-after images of a man with a foot-long pannus and then the same man with six pack abs, and they claim that the diet was responsible for the transformation.

However, the truth is that if we were to take matters into our own hands, we could do that as well without having to spend tens of thousands of dollars on those diets. What must we do, then? Two fundamentals:

- In control of our diet
- Engage in physical activity

Is that too much work right now? Don't we owe that to our body, which has been so helpful to us for so long? We owe it to ourselves and our family, don't we?

This eBook will show you how to improve your life by eating healthfully and generally changing your diet. And we are capable of doing that in a very major way.

CHAPTER 3

What Is the Perfect Diet?

Healthy eating is crucial. You must be aware of the best diet for that.

In actuality, no one can precisely define what an ideal diet is. Now, if you asked someone what a healthy diet is, they might be able to explain it to you. However, you must see the person in question in order to determine their perfect diet. The type of lifestyle a person leads, their age, gender, how much physical activity they get during the day, even their geographic location and temperature, all have a significant impact on their ideal diets.

The first question that needs to be addressed is how many calories each person needs to consume. Naturally, this differs from person to person, primarily based on their amount of physical activity. The following graph illustrates numerous types of people, each with unique characteristics, together with the daily calorie requirements that would make up their perfect diet.

The best diet for each individual varies, however there are some universal principles that hold true for everyone:-

- The diet should have a sufficient amount of carbohydrates, but not too many. Overconsumption of carbohydrates might result in a rise in blood glucose levels.
- Use of fried foods must be kept to a minimum. If at all, there should only be one serving of fried food per day.
- The meal must have green vegetables. Although there are rare exceptions in both directions, the general rule is that foods with better colors are more nutritious. i.e., there are foods without color that are healthy (for instance, cabbage) and there is a large list of foods with color that are unhealthy.
- It's best to choose lean meats. A dinner that is heavy on meat and dairy products but lacking in veggies is particularly unhealthy.
- The amount of cooking should be exactly right while preserving the items' original flavors. Although spices improve the taste of food, they also deplete it of some nutrients, thus they should only be used sparingly.
- It is best to stay away from synthetic fabrics altogether.

CHAPTER 4

Benefits of a Healthy Diet

You have all the inspiration you need right here to continue eating well.

Improves Your Health

Even if we wrote a comprehensive book on the advantages of a healthy diet, it still wouldn't fully cover all of the advantages. The main advantage is that you take charge of your weight.

By eating well, you also ensure that your metabolic processes, particularly your immune and digestive systems, continue to run smoothly. You are also shielded from a number of chronic illnesses, including diabetes and conditions like atherosclerosis and high blood pressure that affect the cardiovascular system.

You'll get More Money

Spend far less money when you eat healthfully. Your grocery bills drop significantly, and if credit card debt is already an issue for you, you avoid adding to it. Additionally, you save a ton of money on any medical costs that may arise as a result of your eating disorder.

Less Dangerous Foods for Your Body

Nowadays, a lot of meals are poisonous due to the synthetic chemicals they contain. One of the fundamental ideas of eating well is that you shouldn't eat anything that is manufactured, so you are far less likely to get these poisons when you are attempting to eat healthy. Additionally, by eating less, you'll be able to cut back on vices like drunkenness and smoking. A beer nearly always signifies a night out with the guys. You won't want the beer if you eat less. Similar to this, you won't want to smoke after every substantial meal like it's a requirement (or more).

Greater Level of Activity

You'll discover that you can perform your work considerably better when you eat better. You can live a more productive life by getting more exercise, traveling, playing, and working. That certainly beats being a slob who spends the entire day vegging out on the couch, don't you think? Your life can be improved by getting more involved with your friends and family.

Improved Social Life

Forget about feederism and the fat fetish; obese people do not have a desirable appearance. The social stigma surrounding carrying extra weight in the incorrect locations on the body is very strong. Your extra weight can actually get in the way of finding a spouse. Not only that, but society despises those who are unable to control their eating behaviors and weight since they are seen as lacking basic self-control. Although not many will discuss it, this type of psychology does exist. You'll discover that these issues go away when you eat well.

How to Lose Weight by Eating Well

A lot of information about eating healthy to lose weight is readily available. However, certain things are more significant than food itself. Let's start with those issues. Your efforts to lose weight would be ineffective without these.

Motivation

Without the correct motivation, no one can successfully reduce weight. You must have a specific objective in mind; this is what keeps you motivated. This objective could be the desire to feel healthier, look better (read: be smaller), be more physically active, or anything else. Then, you must decide to achieve this aim. You must keep this objective in mind. You can map out your path much more effectively when you are certain of the destination.

Support and Motivation

Even if there are people who have lost weight on their own, having family and friends to encourage them makes things much easier. The system will function when they continue to encourage them rather than mock them. Some people have shed pounds solely to improve their ability to contribute to their families.

This can be a very potent emotion and is quite effective for weight loss. If you can participate in a weight loss program alongside another person, it is also highly beneficial. A slight competitive advantage is beneficial. In actuality, rivalry can be beneficial. Nothing is more satisfying than the desire to demonstrate your abilities to someone.

The dietary plan itself is done afterwards.

Now, resist the urge to follow the many food fads you encounter online. These are utterly superfluous. Your own willpower and some effort in making the appropriate eating choices are all you need.It is better to create a detailed health plan and follow it religiously.

One such health program may be found at http://www.joyfullivingservices.com/idealdiet.html

Here is a useful link if you're looking for a child's plan: http://www.vegsource.com/attwood/stages.htm

These diets have a great chance of success, so you won't need a fad diet to support you. You can be your own personal trainer.

CHAPTER 5

It's Not Just About Eating Right

You also require other things to live a full life. Just eating healthfully is insufficient.

You must have heard often how crucial it is to balance your eating habits with a variety of other healthy lifestyle choices in order to improve your quality of life. Though a very significant component of our life, diet is not the sole aspect of who we are. When we talk of a supplement to diet, exercise immediately comes to mind. Exercise is quite important, as we all already know. There will be very little advantage from your newly improved eating habits if you continue to be a couch potato despite eating healthily.

Other things of this nature must be included to our healthy diet and workout routines. Following is a list.

Positive Mentality

A person is more likely to succeed in every area of life if they are perpetually upbeat and enthusiastic about life. The ability to think positively is a crucial component of wellbeing.

CHAPTER 6

Taking Care of the Food, Family, and Friends

When we are attempting to take care of ourselves, we may feel as though we are neglecting our family and friends. The sensation of vanity enters at this point.

When they start a healthy eating diet, many people find that they have to pay far more than they anticipated. I have heard the following things: -

My kids detest me now since I started a natural eating diet for them at home. - A mom of three who stays at home.

"Did I make a mistake? My husband believes that I am more preoccupied with my weight than with him. - A wife of 20 years old.

They believed I wouldn't want the temptation to come my way, so I merely didn't accept an invitation to a party. – a middle-aged man who works in an office.

These events occur naturally. Such events occur after we start a diet plan. The ridicule of those around us must be faced head-on initially. It's true that some individuals will make fun of you if you start a diet. But if we don't start a diet and keep gaining weight, we must keep in mind that there are a lot more individuals who will make fun of us.

The second issue is that someone who is following a healthy eating plan may want other people in their immediate vicinity to do the same. Women will attempt to persuade their family members to adopt a healthier diet, and men will attempt to persuade their friends to adopt a healthier diet. You now need to understand something. Before you were completely convinced of its benefits, not even you were following this healthy eating plan. You didn't begin immediately, did you? You were deliberate. You didn't start taking things more seriously until you realized that you needed to take care of your health. However, you shouldn't anticipate that everyone else would adopt a healthy eating plan as soon as you do. If they choose to continue eating healthfully, they will take their time. Do your best to persuade them by outlining the health advantages and other advantages that starting a healthy diet will bring. However, hold off on forcing them to eat those sprouts just yet.

One further factor is that folks who are following a healthy diet plan often exaggerate how difficult it is. They'll want the public to be aware of the extreme food sacrifices they're making. They will boast to everyone about skipping meals and consuming only wholesome foods, etc. However, doing this can exclude you from some social groups. For instance, your pals might forget to call you the next time they visit Taco Bell. The best course of action would be to tell your pals that you occasionally let your hair down, which is truly what you need to do to avoid stress. They won't be too concerned about your eating habits if you do this.

CHAPTER 7

Your Motives for Eating Healthily

Whatever you undertake, you need to have the correct motivation. This is especially true if you're trying to start a challenging healthy eating regimen.

Most people find it challenging to start a healthy eating routine. You've been chowing down on fried meals and downing cokes and beers for so long that the thought of giving them all up can be terrifying. In reality, this phobia around dieting prevents the majority of individuals from considering eating healthily. They don't believe they can make it through it. Of course, you don't have to be so painful on yourself straight away. Start slowly and eliminate one food group at a time.

If you can cut back on the amount and frequency of your meals, you don't necessarily need to quit eating altogether. As an alternative, you may eat well during the week and indulge in a small feast one weekend. There are a few ways to circumvent the restrictions of healthy eating, but people still want incentive.

Always Remember Your End Goal

Your motivation will increase as the strength of your aim increases. This objective could be anything, such as improving your appearance before a social function, feeling better, becoming more active and energetic, doing activities that your weight prevents you from doing, maintaining your healthy lifestyle, or simply wanting to prove a buddy wrong. The most crucial thing is to firmly remember your objective and then use it as your motivational force.

Make A Decision Not To Give Up

It will be more difficult for you to stray from your healthy eating routine if you create a resolution that you won't break. If at all feasible, make this decision in front of your loved ones, close friends, or coworkers. This is beneficial since it will help you recall your resolution whenever you are tempted to eat something unhealthy and resist.

Choose a Difficult Activity

Try to pique your interest in something that is challenging for you right now but will get easier if your body is in better shape. Dance and swimming are both excellent options. If you give these things a try, they can keep you quite interested, but you'll need to get in better shape to accomplish them successfully. The best thing is that you naturally lose weight when you dance or go swimming!

Choose a Partner

The best motivation you could find is this. Invite a companion to begin the healthy eating regimen with you if they are experiencing a similar issue. You two will be fantastic motivators for one another. You two could even compete against one another to see who does better. This is beneficial because you have company and are not on this mission by yourself.

CHAPTER 8
How to Avoid Becoming Obsessed with Eating Right

We need to eat well, but how well? What is the limit of this?

While eating healthfully is vital, it's equally crucial to avoid obsessing over it. The issues start at that point.

Obsession with healthy eating may cause a number of issues. You can have multiple instances of excessive stress. A hormone called cortisol is released when you feel anxious. The body suffers as a result of this. The body's metabolic functions are slowed down by cortisol, which significantly worsens the weight issue.

This is only one of the many reasons you shouldn't become fixated on healthy eating. Another issue is that by severely limiting your food intake, you might be depriving your body of the necessary amount of nutrition. Your body may not be getting the vitamins it needs to grow properly, which could cause dietary deficiency disorders to become an issue for you. Additionally, malnutrition can lead to anorexia, a condition that can lead to a full Pandora's Box of health issues.

The social component is the next thing to think about. You might be torturing other people with your food obsessions, whether knowingly or unknowingly, as we've already seen.

Therefore, it's crucial that you don't take your healthy eating habit too far and turn it into an obsession. Don't let it dictate your life; you are doing this to handle it.

Treating yourself occasionally is the best course of action. On that particular day of the week, indulge yourself. Bring your family with you. This meal might be served on Sunday. Your family will now be aware that you are allowed to eat anything on this day. Enjoy a wonderful lunch that day, largely as a treat for sticking with it all week. In fact, if you approach this in the correct way, every Sunday can end up being a celebration for you.

It won't become an obsession if you don't overstress.

You can utilize a variety of breathing and mind-control techniques. Along with your physical health, take care of your mind. The easiest method to stop stress from destroying your mental space is to do this. These exercises can be learned from a variety of fitness programs that are shown on television as well as from a number of videos on websites like YouTube.

CHAPTER 9

Healthy Eating And Life Management

You'll notice that after eating healthfully for a while, things start to fall into place on their own. Your life drastically improves all of a sudden, and you start to realize that you are taking back control. And the reason for all of this is because you are now in charge of your eating habits.

The most crucial aspect is that you must maintain your motivation. Probably since you were overweight when you started, you followed a "eat right" plan. You've now overcame that predicament thanks to your consistent efforts. Your physical condition has greatly improved. But that doesn't imply you can start overindulging right away. You must keep up your healthy eating routine. You won't start to feel its actual impact in controlling your life until that time.

A two-month commitment to a healthy eating plan will result in lifelong adherence. This is true. Therefore, you only need to maintain your attention for those two months. You'll discover that the advantages you experience throughout those two months will keep you devoted to the program for life.

Find instances and examples of people who have brought their lives under control by controlling their eating habits by reading books, watching videos, conducting Internet research, or watching videos. These stories will inspire you greatly, and you will want to apply them to your own life.

So, continue. Eating well is the best course of action if you want to enhance your ability to manage physical duties, increase your stamina, or simply lose some unwanted weight. All of these advantages will be available to you, but maybe most importantly, you will be able to spend more time with your loved ones. If nothing else, this is what will genuinely assist you in controlling and enriching your life.

Conclusion

It is up to you to run your life. One of the finest approaches is to eat healthily. What that means to you is now clear to you.

Make a plan for a nutritious diet for yourself right away.

Best wishes for you!

www.ingramcontent.com/pod-product-compliance
Lightning Source LLC
LaVergne TN
LVHW012034160826
845678LV00013B/2597